Comprehensive Guide to Rheumatoid Arthritis

Understanding Causes, Symptoms, Treatment Options and Clinical Implications – A Must-Have Handbook for Patients and Caregivers
(Things You Must Know)

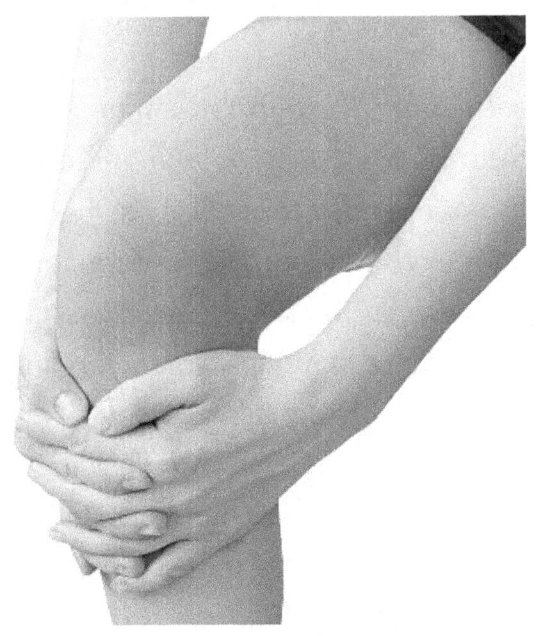

By

Isabella White

Copyright © 2024 by Isabella White.

Table of Contents

Introduction

Rheumatoid arthritis (RA) is a chronic autoimmune disease characterized by painful inflammation and eventual damage to the joints. It is one of the most common types of arthritis, affecting over 1.3 million adults in the United States and nearly 1% of the global population. While rheumatoid arthritis can develop at any age, its onset most commonly occurs between 30 and 60. Women are up to three times more likely to develop the disease than men.

Rheumatoid arthritis is an autoimmune condition resulting from the body's immune system mistakenly attacking healthy tissue. In RA, the immune system targets the synovium, a thin membrane that lines the joints. This causes thickening and inflammation of the synovium, eventually destroying cartilage and bone within the joints. Over time, the inflammation and damage can lead to deformity and disability if left untreated.

The most commonly affected joints are the smaller joints of the hands and feet and the wrists, elbows, shoulders, knees, ankles, and hips. Symptoms typically develop slowly over weeks or months. They include joint pain, swelling, stiffness, and loss of function. RA often starts gradually with minor symptoms like fatigue and general aches before progressing to more severe joint symptoms.

While the exact causes of RA are not fully understood, a combination of genetic and environmental factors is believed to play a role. Genetic factors make some individuals more susceptible to developing an abnormal immune response. Potential environmental triggers include smoking, infections, and hormonal changes.

There is no cure for rheumatoid arthritis, but early diagnosis and proper treatment can help minimize joint damage and allow patients to manage their symptoms. Treatment focuses on controlling inflammation, relieving pain, slowing disease progression, and improving quality of life. Medications, physical therapy, exercise, joint protection techniques, and sometimes surgery are utilized.

Rheumatoid arthritis can significantly impact a person's daily life. Patients face physical limitations and disability, an increased risk of depression and cardiovascular disease, and socioeconomic challenges. However, with comprehensive management focused on treating the disease and its symptoms, many patients can find ways to continue enjoying active, fulfilling lives.

The Purpose and Scope of the Book

This book serves as a comprehensive, patient-focused guide to understanding rheumatoid arthritis and the array of treatment options and lifestyle impacts associated with the disease. It aims to empower rheumatoid arthritis patients, as well as their caregivers and loved ones, with the knowledge needed to take control of managing this chronic inflammatory condition.

Within these pages, readers will gain a deeper understanding of the signs, symptoms, causes, risk factors, diagnosis, and available treatments for rheumatoid arthritis. The book explores pharmacological treatments such as DMARDs, biologics, steroids, pain medications, and non-drug approaches, including physical therapy, joint protection techniques, exercise regimens, massage, and mindfulness. Surgical options are also discussed.

In addition to exploring treatments, the book provides practical advice for living with rheumatoid arthritis day-to-day. It offers tips and strategies for managing pain, fatigue, mobility challenges, and common daily activities. Recommendations for workplace accommodations, assistive devices, and protecting joints are included. The psychosocial aspects of coping with a chronic illness are also addressed.

This handbook aims to prepare readers to have informed discussions with their healthcare providers regarding treatment options and disease management. It equips patients and caregivers with questions to ask their doctor and a framework for evaluating treatments and lifestyle changes. The goal is to help readers become active, engaged participants in their care.

While this book provides a comprehensive overview of rheumatoid arthritis, it does not replace professional medical advice. Readers should consult a licensed rheumatologist or primary care physician for guidance on specific treatment plans and recommendations tailored to their health status and needs.

The expansive scope of this guide makes it suitable for those newly diagnosed with rheumatoid arthritis and those living long-term with the disease. Patients of all ages and backgrounds can benefit from enhancing their knowledge about this condition. Caregivers, loved ones, and family members can use this handbook to understand rheumatoid arthritis better and learn how to support someone with it.

With the information in this all-encompassing guide, rheumatoid arthritis patients and their support systems will feel empowered, prepared, and equipped to navigate life with this challenging chronic illness. Knowledge lays the foundation for taking control of rheumatoid arthritis rather than letting it control you.

Chapter 1

Understanding Rheumatoid Arthritis

Rheumatoid Arthritis as an Inflammatory and Autoimmune Disease

Rheumatoid arthritis (RA) is classified as an inflammatory autoimmune disease. This means it involves chronic inflammation caused by the body's immune system mistakenly attacking healthy tissue.

In autoimmune diseases like rheumatoid arthritis, the immune system fails to properly distinguish between foreign invaders that could cause harm and the body's healthy cells or tissues. The immune system contains specialized white blood cells that normally identify and neutralize viruses, bacteria, and other potentially dangerous foreign substances called antigens. However, immune cells cannot differentiate between antigens and healthy tissue in autoimmune conditions. They launch an immune response against the body's cells or tissues as if they were harmful invaders.

In rheumatoid arthritis, this abnormal autoimmune attack targets the synovium membranes that line the joints. The synovium produces synovial fluid, which acts as a lubricant to nourish joint cartilage and tissues. When the immune cells attack the synovium, inflammation flares up in the joint linings. This causes painful swelling, stiffness, and loss of function in the joints that characterize rheumatoid arthritis.

Several types of immune cells are involved in this inflammatory attack on the joints. T-cells and B-cells, two key components of the immune system, are believed to play central roles in the development and progression of rheumatoid arthritis. However, the exact trigger for this misdirected immune response remains unknown. Researchers continue investigating potential genetic, hormonal, and environmental factors that could disrupt the immune balance and set off rheumatoid arthritis.

Left unchecked, the chronic inflammation of RA can eventually destroy cartilage and bone within the joints. The inflamed synovium grows abnormally thick and can invade and erode nearby cartilage and bone. It also secretes enzymes and acids that break down the tissues inside the joint capsule. Over months and years, the joint damage leads to increasing pain, stiffness, deformity, and disability.

The inflammation caused by rheumatoid arthritis also impacts the whole body, not just the joints. It can contribute to fever, appetite loss, and weight changes. Rheumatoid arthritis inflammation puts patients at higher risk of cardiovascular disease and osteoporosis as well. Managing inflammation is crucial to relieve joint symptoms and reduce the risk of systemic complications.

Because rheumatoid arthritis is driven by inflammation from an overactive, confused immune system, treatments aim to suppress this abnormal autoimmune response and minimize joint damage. A better understanding of the inflammatory-autoimmune nature of RA helps patients and doctors determine the most suitable therapies.

Prevalence, Incidence Rates, and Age/Gender Distribution of Rheumatoid Arthritis Globally

Rheumatoid arthritis (RA) impacts over 1.3 million adults in the United States. Approximately 0.6% of the overall U.S. adult population suffers from rheumatoid arthritis. The worldwide prevalence is estimated to be around 0.24%, meaning about 1 in every 400–500 individuals globally have rheumatoid arthritis.

Each year in the U.S., there are over 41 new cases of rheumatoid arthritis per 100,000 people. Rheumatoid arthritis affects all ethnic and racial groups. However, some populations have higher incidence rates, such as certain Native American tribes, where 5–8% of the population is affected.

The onset of rheumatoid arthritis typically occurs between ages 30 and 60. The average age of diagnosis is 42 for men and 44 for women. Juvenile rheumatoid arthritis impacts around 1 in 1000 children under the age of 16. After age 80, the incidence of rheumatoid arthritis begins to decline.

Rheumatoid arthritis is 2–3 times more prevalent in women than men. Around 75% of U.S. adults with rheumatoid arthritis are female. Researchers believe sex hormones may play a role in the immune system dysfunction underlying rheumatoid arthritis, which could help explain the higher prevalence in women. The incidence rate among women before age 45 is 2–3 times higher than in men of the same age. After 45, the gap in incidence narrows due to changes in hormone levels.

While rheumatoid arthritis can develop at any age, there are two peak incidence ranges. The first peak occurs between ages 30 and 50, often corresponding to the childbearing years. A secondary peak period emerges around age 75. This pattern suggests a link between hormonal changes and rheumatoid arthritis risk across the lifespan.

Besides gender and age, family history is another strong risk factor. If a first-degree relative, like a sibling or parent, has rheumatoid arthritis, one's risk is 3 to 5 times higher. This supports a genetic component in addition to environmental triggers. Rheumatoid arthritis does not seem directly inherited, but certain genes increase susceptibility. The shared HLA genetic marker is found in most RA patients.

Geographic location also impacts rheumatoid arthritis incidence. Rates are lower near the equator and increase further away in both the Northern and Southern hemispheres. This points to possible environmental influences like vitamin D from sunlight exposure. Urban populations exhibit higher rates than rural ones.

In the U.S., there are differences in rheumatoid arthritis prevalence across ethnic groups, according to CDC data. Native Americans have the highest prevalence at 6.8%, followed by Caucasians at 4.2%,

Hispanics at 2.6%, Asians at 2%, and African-Americans at 1.6%. Understanding distribution statistics helps inform research on RA risk factors.

Tracking incidence rates also enables the projection of the growing population with rheumatoid arthritis as life expectancies rise. While prevalence fluctuates by subgroup, rheumatoid arthritis remains a significant global health issue, affecting around 1% of adults worldwide. Ongoing research strives to uncover why certain individuals develop rheumatoid arthritis in hopes of improving prevention, diagnosis, and treatment.

Risk Factors and Potential Causes

The exact causes of rheumatoid arthritis are not yet fully understood, but research indicates that genetic and environmental factors play important roles. While rheumatoid arthritis is not directly inherited, genetic makeup does influence a person's susceptibility. Environmental triggers are likely needed to initiate the autoimmune attack on joints in those with genetic predispositions.

Studies of twins provide insight into the genetic link. Identical twins share nearly 100% of the same genes. If one twin has rheumatoid arthritis, the other has a 15–30% chance of developing the disease, too. For non-identical twins, who share only about 50% of genes, the risk drops to 5% if one twin has rheumatoid arthritis. This shows that a genetic component exists.

Certain gene mutations affecting the immune system are more common in those with rheumatoid arthritis. The shared epitope HLA-DRB1 gene is present in up to 70% of rheumatoid arthritis patients but only 30% of the general public. Researchers believe this shared epitope may allow cells to present proteins to the immune system in a way that triggers an abnormal autoimmune response. Hundreds of other genes likely contribute to varying degrees as well.

While genetics set the stage, external environmental factors often act as the triggers to initiate rheumatoid arthritis. These include:

1. **Smoking:** Smoking cigarettes is the top environmental risk factor, nearly doubling the risk of developing rheumatoid arthritis. Quitting smoking can lower the risk.

2. **Infections:** Certain viral or bacterial infections are suspected triggers, especially in those with genetic predispositions. Epstein-Barr virus, hepatitis C, mycoplasma, and chlamydia infections may play a role.

3. **Hormones:** Rheumatoid arthritis is 2-3 times more common in women, pointing to hormones like estrogen or progesterone influencing risk. Oral contraceptives and hormone therapy have also been loosely implicated.

4. **Obesity:** Carrying excess weight has been associated with an increased risk of developing rheumatoid arthritis due to factors like chronic inflammation.

5. **Environmental pollutants:** Air pollution, pesticides, and other industrial chemicals may act as environmental triggers for sensitive individuals.

6. **Stress:** Emotional or physical stress may worsen rheumatoid arthritis by stimulating inflammatory responses. The link to developing RA needs to be clarified.

7. **Diet:** Some dietary factors, like low antioxidants, vitamin D deficiency, and high salt intake, may raise susceptibility, but more research is needed.

8. **Periodontal disease:** Bacteria involved in gum disease might trigger autoimmunity in susceptible people. Managing periodontal disease may lower the risk.

The influence of these environmental exposures likely depends on the person's unique genetic makeup. Ongoing research aims to clarify how potential risk factors interact with genes to initiate the onset of rheumatoid arthritis.

Identifying the triggers that cause the immune system to malfunction can aid prevention efforts and early detection. While not all risks are avoidable, knowledge allows patients to lower modifiable risks where possible through lifestyle approaches.

Pathophysiology and Role of the Immune System and Inflammation

In rheumatoid arthritis, the immune system wrongly attacks the body's tissues, specifically the joints' synovial membranes. This triggers chronic inflammation, joint damage, and the painful symptoms of RA. Understanding the immune factors and inflammatory processes underlying this autoimmune pathology provides insight into disease progression and treatment.

Normal immune function involves various cells and proteins working together to identify and target foreign invaders, like viruses and bacteria, without reacting to healthy cells. In autoimmune diseases like rheumatoid arthritis, this ability to distinguish oneself from others fails.

Researchers believe genetics and environmental triggers contribute to the immune system malfunction in rheumatoid arthritis. Genetic susceptibility factors and exposures like infections or hormones disrupt the immune balance and create an abnormal inflammatory cascade.

Once triggered, the immune attack centers around the synovium, or synovial membrane, in joints. The synovium produces synovial fluid to nourish joint tissues. In rheumatoid arthritis, immune system T-cells mistakenly identify synovium proteins as harmful antigens and launch an assault.

Activated T-cells recruit other immune cells, like B-cells, macrophages, and cytokines, to join the attack. Cytokines are small proteins vital for cell signaling and regulating immune responses. In rheumatoid arthritis, pro-inflammatory cytokines like tumor necrosis factor-alpha (TNF-α), interleukin-1 (IL-1), and interleukin-6 (IL-6) stimulate rampant inflammation.

As more immune cells flood the joint synovium, inflammation flares up. The synovium grows abnormally thicker, invading and eroding nearby cartilage and bone. Enzymes secreted by the inflamed synovium break down collagen in the cartilage and bone.

Chronic inflammation also triggers pain receptors, increasing joint pain and tenderness. Swelling results as excess fluid accumulates and the joint stiffens up. Over time, the progressive joint destruction leads to deformity, disability, and chronic pain.

This immune-driven inflammatory process not only affects joints but can also contribute to systemic issues like cardiovascular disease, lung damage, depression, fatigue, and osteoporosis. Managing inflammation is key to preventing irreversible joint erosion and organ damage.

Understanding the pathological sequence helps explain why medications that suppress the immune response or inhibit inflammatory proteins often successfully alleviate rheumatoid arthritis symptoms and progression. Biologic drugs like TNF inhibitors block pro-inflammatory cytokines that drive inflammation. Early intensive treatment to halt inflammation can limit joint damage.

While the exact immune triggers for rheumatoid arthritis remain uncertain, insight into the resulting inflammatory cascade informs approaches for slowing disease progression, maintaining joint health, and improving patient quality of life.

Chapter 2

Signs and Symptoms

Common Initial Symptoms of RA

In the early stages of rheumatoid arthritis, symptoms tend to develop gradually for weeks or months. The most characteristic initial symptoms include joint pain, swelling, stiffness, and fatigue.

Joint pain is often one of the first noticeable rheumatoid arthritis symptoms. It typically begins slowly as a vague ache or tenderness affecting a few joints, especially in the smaller joints of the hands and feet. This early joint pain often has a symmetrical pattern, meaning it impacts the same joints on both sides of the body—both wrists or both sides of the fingers, for example.

The joint pain usually worsens with movement and improves with rest. It often follows a cyclical pattern, flaring up for weeks or months, then subsiding for a time before recurring. Morning joint stiffness lasting over 30 minutes is common. The pain and stiffness tend to increase in severity over time.

Joint swelling results as synovial fluid accumulates in the inflamed joints. The swelling often coincides with or follows joint pain. It may cause the joints or fingers to appear puffy or distorted. The swelling can range from mild to quite pronounced in some cases.

Muscle and joint stiffness are other hallmark rheumatoid arthritis symptoms that emerge early on. The stiffness tends to be most severe during the morning or after prolonged sitting. It can make it difficult for basic movements like standing up, walking, gripping objects, or getting dressed—stiffness lasting over an hour in the morning points to possible rheumatoid arthritis.

In addition to joint symptoms, increased fatigue often accompanies early rheumatoid arthritis. Patients may notice a lack of energy, exhaustion, or feeling unwell, even with adequate rest. Fatigue results from the inflammatory processes and immune activity happening throughout the body.

Other non-specific symptoms like occasional fevers, appetite changes leading to weight loss, firm lumps (rheumatoid nodules) under the skin, eye dryness or pain, and tingling in the fingers or feet can also manifest in the early stages but are less common.

Early rheumatoid arthritis symptoms frequently come and go and may even resolve temporarily before recurring again. Since the symptoms mimic those of other conditions like osteoarthritis or age-related joint pain, rheumatoid arthritis often goes undiagnosed initially.

Catching the distinct symptoms early and recognizing the progressive pattern over time allows for prompt diagnosis and treatment to prevent irreversible joint damage. Ongoing monitoring of symptoms provides helpful information to doctors when making diagnoses and tailoring treatment plans. Paying attention to even subtle symptom changes is key.

The Progression of Rheumatoid Arthritis Symptoms If Left Untreated

Without treatment, rheumatoid arthritis symptoms tend to worsen over time and lead to increased disability and joint damage. Early inflammatory changes in the joints become more pronounced and widespread as the immune system's attack persists unabated.

In the first few months after onset, symptoms like joint pain, stiffness, and fatigue fluctuate in severity but may briefly disappear with stretches. Over time, the symptom-free periods disappear as inflammation causes ongoing irreversible joint changes.

The joint pain becomes more constant and severe rather than intermittent. Even at rest, patients experience throbbing joint pain. The pain worsens with movement or weight-bearing on joints. More joints beyond the hands and feet, including the knees, shoulders, elbows, hips, and neck, are affected.

Joint stiffness lasts longer each morning and becomes more debilitating. Simple tasks require extensive limbering up of stiff, painful joints—joint swelling and deformity increase, with abnormal growths damaging the joint structure. Joints can take on misshapen appearances.

Fatigue from immune activity often prevents patients from getting adequate activity and sleep. Severe fatigue and flu-like malaise may occur. Appetite diminishes due to proteins secreted by the immune system, leading to unintended weight loss.

Without medications to halt disease progression, inflammatory molecules destroy cartilage, bone, and soft tissues inside the joints. This leads to irreversible joint damage and erosion. Joints lose integrity and stability, becoming prone to deformity and dislocation.

The range of motion in the joints diminishes as scarring and erosion limit mobility. Activities requiring gripping, lifting, twisting, bending, or reaching become increasingly challenging. Disability and reliance on assistive devices or the help of others for daily tasks often result.

In advanced rheumatoid arthritis, chronic inflammation can cause ruptured tendons and soft tissue nodules under the skin. In severe cases, joints may dislocate or fuse in fixed, misaligned positions. The wrists, metacarpophalangeal joints in the hands, and cervical spine are especially prone to instability and structural damage.

Over the years, patients experience a gradual loss of joint function and increasing pain with no remission. Remodeling of joint bones causes severely deformed and dysfunctional joints, leaving patients disabled without surgery or joint replacements.

Extra-articular symptoms may also emerge as inflammation damages tissues like the heart, lungs, blood vessels, nerves, and eyes. These complications increase the risks of heart attack, stroke, infections, lymphoma, and blindness.

Early diagnosis and treatment are critical to preventing the rapid progression of joint damage and disability associated with rheumatoid arthritis. Medications to control inflammation and suppress the immune system response can effectively minimize symptoms, reduce future joint damage, and maintain day-to-day function when started promptly.

Joint Damage and Deformities That Can Occur in Advanced Rheumatoid Arthritis

Without adequate treatment, the inflammatory processes of rheumatoid arthritis can lead to progressively worsening joint damage, deformity, and disability. Nearly any joint can be impacted, but the hands and wrists are most vulnerable to disfiguring changes.

In the hands, rheumatoid arthritis frequently causes instabilities and drifts in the metacarpophalangeal (MCP) and proximal interphalangeal (PIP) finger joints. Ligaments stretch and rupture, allowing the finger joints to displace and deviate.

Swan neck deformities can occur in the fingers, characterized by hyperextension of the PIP joint and flexion of the DIP joint into a bent position resembling a swan's neck. The drifts and ligament instability enable the abnormal positioning.

Over time, the MCP joints also move to the side, called ulnar drift. This happens because synovial proliferation causes the joint capsules and ligaments to stretch. Fingers take on a zig-zag appearance as the bone ends gradually dislocate.

Boutonnière deformities affecting the PIP joints are another common occurrence, causing the joints to be fixed in flexion. Tendons snap over the dislocated bones, blocking full extension. This leads to a claw-like finger posture.

In the wrists, carpal collapse alters the normal anatomical alignment into a severe deformity. The row of small carpal bones slumps downward, with a deviation of the hand to the ulnar (pinky finger) side. Wrists are prone to instability and frequent dislocation.

Erosive changes in the finger and wrist bones can cause rapidly progressing joint damage and bone loss. The inflamed synovium invades and destroys the bone ends, causing pitting and full-thickness erosions detectable on X-rays.

The forefoot may take on a flattened appearance in the feet with the loss of the transverse arch. Joint instability enables abnormal side-to-side motion. Pressure points lead to calluses and ulcers on the feet.

The cervical spine (neck) is also often affected, especially the atlantoaxial joint connecting the C1 and C2 vertebrae. Ligament damage leads to instability, subluxation injuries, and spinal cord compression. Spinal fractures can result.

Other common areas impacted include the shoulders, elbows, knees, and hips. Muscular atrophy around affected joints exacerbates mobility limitations and weakness. Joint replacements may be necessary to restore function in severely damaged joints.

While joint damage varies by individual, ongoing inflammation inevitably takes a toll if not adequately controlled with medications. Early diagnosis and treatment are key to limiting irreversible joint changes and preserving mobility and function.

Even with therapy, some residual joint abnormalities and fragility persist. Patients must learn adaptive techniques through daily movements and activities to protect vulnerable joints and prevent further damage. With vigilance and tailored treatment, progression can be minimized.

Extra-Articular Manifestations of Rheumatoid Arthritis

In addition to joint symptoms, rheumatoid arthritis can lead to extra-articular manifestations that impact other tissues and organ systems. These complications result from chronic inflammation and immune activity. Common extra-articular manifestations include rheumatoid nodules, Sjögren's syndrome, lung disease, and cardiovascular disease.

Rheumatoid nodules are benign, firm lumps that form under the skin, often near affected joints. They range from pea-sized to several centimeters large, and develop in about 20% of rheumatoid arthritis patients. Nodules frequently form on the elbows, hands, and feet. While usually painless, they can sometimes become inflamed or infected.

Sjögren's syndrome co-occurs in about 15% of rheumatoid arthritis patients. It causes inflammation and dysfunction of the tear and salivary glands. Symptoms include dry eyes, mouth, throat, and skin. If untreated can lead to eye damage, dental decay, and skin fragility.

Lung complications like pleuritis, rheumatoid lung nodules, and interstitial lung disease affect up to 10% of rheumatoid arthritis patients. Inflammation of lung tissues leads to chest pain, shortness of breath, coughing, and increased respiratory infections.

Up to half of rheumatoid arthritis patients develop some degree of cardiovascular disease. Chronic inflammation promotes atherosclerosis, raising the risk of heart attack and stroke. Pericarditis, or sac inflammation surrounding the heart, can also occur.

Peripheral neuropathy, causing numbness and tingling in the extremities, affects nearly one-third of patients. Carpal tunnel syndrome, resulting from inflamed wrist tendons, frequently necessitates surgery.

Inflammation in blood vessels (vasculitis) leads to skin rashes and leg ulcers. Dry eyes and mouth occur as tears and saliva glands are impacted. Anemia arises from impaired red blood cell production.

Due to pro-inflammatory molecules, osteoporosis speeds up bone loss, particularly in the hip and spine. Vertebral fractures and hip fractures are concerns.

While joint symptoms are most pronounced, managing extra-articular inflammation and complications is key to preserving overall health. Rheumatoid arthritis therapies like DMARDs that reduce whole-body inflammation help minimize the risk of organ damage. Early detection allows for prompt intervention.

Chapter 3

Getting a Diagnosis

Diagnostic Criteria and Tests

Diagnosing rheumatoid arthritis involves a combination of physical examination findings, imaging tests, and laboratory tests. No single test can definitively confirm a diagnosis, so physicians synthesize multiple sources of information to determine if criteria for rheumatoid arthritis are met.

A physical examination allows doctors to check for key signs like swollen, tender joints, stiffness and reduced range of motion, nodules under the skin, warmth or redness over joints, and alignment changes or deformities. While not specific to RA, these findings provide clues.

Imaging tests like X-rays, ultrasounds, and MRI scans visualize joint structures and damage. X-rays reveal loss of bone density, areas of bone erosion, and joint alignment changes over time. Ultrasounds and MRIs detect early fluid accumulation, synovial thickening, and cartilage loss before changes appear on X-rays.

Lab tests check for elevated levels of RF or anti-CCP antibodies in the blood. Rheumatoid factor (RF) antibodies are present in about 70–80% of rheumatoid arthritis patients. However, RF can also occur in other conditions. Anti-cyclic citrullinated peptide (anti-CCP) antibodies are more specific to rheumatoid arthritis.

Other lab work involves complete blood counts, ESR/CRP levels, and joint fluid analysis. Anemia and elevated inflammatory markers provide supporting evidence of rheumatoid arthritis. Doctors may analyze joint fluid for signs of inflammation.

Current diagnostic criteria for rheumatoid arthritis require:

- Confirmed presence of synovitis (swollen, inflamed joints) in at least one joint
- Testing positive for RF or anti-CCP antibodies
- Signs and symptoms lasting over six weeks

Additionally, other potential causes like lupus, gout, psoriatic arthritis, and osteoarthritis must be ruled out. Doctors also assess the number and pattern of affected joints and the impact on daily function.

No single test or set of criteria confirms rheumatoid arthritis. The diagnosis integrates clinical, laboratory, and imaging information tailored to the patient's presentation. Other conditions, like viral infections, can mimic rheumatoid arthritis symptoms, so ongoing monitoring helps confirm the diagnosis.

Early diagnosis is crucial for starting treatment promptly to prevent rapid joint damage. Patients who present with at least three affected joints, morning stiffness over an hour, elevated inflammatory markers, and high RF/anti-CCP titers can be diagnosed definitively based on strong probability, even if criteria are not fully met yet.

After diagnosis, regular follow-up appointments monitor disease progression through physical exams, blood tests for inflammatory markers, and repeat imaging. Checking that treatment effectively manages inflammation and prevents further joint damage is essential to ongoing rheumatoid arthritis care.

The Role of RF, Anti-CCP, ESR, and CRP in Diagnosing Rheumatoid Arthritis

Certain blood tests are frequently used to aid in diagnosing rheumatoid arthritis and monitoring disease progression. Some of these tests are for rheumatoid factor (RF), anti-cyclic citrullinated peptide (anti-CCP) antibodies, erythrocyte sedimentation rate (ESR), and C-reactive protein (CRP).

Rheumatoid factor is an antibody detected through a blood test in about 70–80% of rheumatoid arthritis patients. It is often one of the first abnormal lab results indicating potential RA. However, RF is not specific to rheumatoid arthritis. It can also occur in other inflammatory conditions or sometimes even in healthy older adults.

Anti-CCP antibodies are antibodies that react to citrullinated proteins in the joints. The anti-CCP blood test checks for these particular antibodies and is more specific for confirming a rheumatoid arthritis diagnosis. Around 50–80% of RA patients test positive for anti-CCP, while only 1–3% of healthy adults exhibit these antibodies.

The presence of either RF or anti-CCP antibodies, especially at high levels, supports a rheumatoid arthritis diagnosis when consistent with clinical presentation. However, negative RF or anti-CCP results do not rule out RA, as some patients test negative. Doctors interpret results in combination with other factors.

ESR (erythrocyte sedimentation rate) and CRP (C-reactive protein) measure levels of inflammatory markers in the blood. Active inflammation causes elevated ESR and CRP. These tests help assess the level of disease activity in rheumatoid arthritis patients.

ESR measures how quickly red blood cells settle at the bottom of a test tube over one hour. Faster settling indicates excess proteins from inflammation. CRP directly quantifies levels of the C-reactive protein biomarker released by inflamed tissues.

Monitoring ESR and CRP over time helps determine if treatment effectively controls rheumatoid arthritis inflammation and flare-ups. Sudden spikes suggest a disease flare. Stable, low levels indicate remission. However, some patients have persistently normal ESR/CRP despite active joint damage, so other measures are still needed.

In newly presenting patients, very high ESR and CRP, along with multiple swollen joints, increase the likelihood of rheumatoid arthritis before other criteria are fully met. These markers can detect inflammatory disease activity even when symptoms are mild. However, by themselves, they do not confirm an RA diagnosis.

In summary, RF, anti-CCP, ESR, and CRP are helpful lab tests supporting evidence in rheumatoid arthritis diagnosis and management. However, the results must be interpreted within the entire clinical context of each patient's condition. A combination of physical exam findings, imaging, and labs determines diagnosis and monitors disease status.

How Doctors Differentiate Rheumatoid Arthritis from Other Types of Arthritis

Rheumatoid arthritis shares features with several other common types, including osteoarthritis, psoriatic arthritis, and gout. Distinguishing rheumatoid arthritis from these other arthritic conditions is important for appropriate treatment.

Osteoarthritis most often affects the hands, knees, hips, and spine. Unlike the symmetrical joint involvement of rheumatoid arthritis, osteoarthritis typically impacts just one or a few joints. It stems from mechanical wear and tear on joints, not autoimmunity. Diagnostic clues include an older age of onset, bony knobs at joint margins, and minimal inflammation without prolonged morning joint stiffness.

Psoriatic arthritis occurs in up to 30% of people with the skin condition psoriasis. Skin patches, pitting nail changes, and negative RF blood tests point toward psoriatic rather than rheumatoid arthritis. Psoriatic arthritis also tends to affect the distal joints of fingers and toes rather than the typically involved joints of rheumatoid arthritis.

Gout causes extremely painful flares of hot, swollen, red joints, most often in the big toe, ankles, or knees. While gout can mimic rheumatoid arthritis symptoms during flares, the intermittent nature and presence of uric acid crystals in joint fluid distinguish it from RA. Blood tests reveal high uric acid levels in gout.

Reactive arthritis secondary to intestinal or genitourinary infections causes asymmetric oligoarticular joint pain, commonly in the lower extremities. Unlike RA, it arises after the precipitating infection and tends to be short-lived. Blood tests are typically negative.

Lyme disease may induce brief arthritis with swelling and pain around one or a few large joints, especially the knee. A history of tick exposure and the circular rash of Lyme disease differentiate it from rheumatoid arthritis. Lyme testing can confirm the diagnosis.

Lupus can also cause arthralgias and arthritis, along with distinct systemic symptoms like the butterfly facial rash and photosensitivity. Blood tests reveal specific autoantibodies, unlike those found in rheumatoid arthritis.

While joint pain is common in numerous arthritic conditions, certain key features help distinguish rheumatoid arthritis. These include a symmetrical pattern of joint involvement, prolonged morning stiffness, elevated inflammatory markers, autoantibodies, and an insidious onset over weeks to months. Considering the whole clinical picture narrows the diagnosis.

Chapter 4

Treatment Options

The Goals of Rheumatoid Arthritis Treatment

The overarching goals of rheumatoid arthritis treatment are to relieve symptoms, stop or slow joint damage, prevent disability, and induce remission so patients can maintain the highest possible quality of life.

Immediate relief of symptoms like pain, stiffness, and fatigue benefits patients' daily experience living with rheumatoid arthritis. Treatment aims to minimize symptomatic flares, make symptoms more tolerable, and restore functional ability. Medications, physical therapy, and lifestyle approaches help ease symptoms.

Preventing further joint damage and erosion is another pivotal treatment goal. Early, aggressive therapy to control inflammation and halt the immune system attack on joints can limit deformities and disabilities down the road. Medications like DMARDs that modify disease progression are key for preserving joint integrity over time.

Maintaining day-to-day physical function and independence are also important goals guiding treatment. If needed, approaches like occupational therapy, custom braces, ambulatory devices, and surgery allow patients to perform daily activities despite joint limitations. The treatment team helps set realistic functional goals.

Inducing a complete or partial remission is ideal to allow patients a prolonged respite from active disease. Remission refers to minimal disease activity causing little to no symptoms. It is associated with a halted progression of joint damage. Remission is more likely with early treatment.

Treatment is highly individualized for each patient's rheumatoid arthritis pattern, symptoms, age, disease severity, and lifestyle. The benefits of reduced symptoms and joint damage must be weighed against potential medication side effects.

Ideally, treatment leads to sustained low disease activity or remission. Flares should become shorter, milder, and farther between. Joint deterioration stabilizes rather than progressing. Patients experience manageable symptoms with minimal lifestyle disruption.

However, rheumatoid arthritis waxes and wanes over a lifetime. Periodic flares are expected. The treatment focus during flares is returning to baseline levels of symptoms and functioning promptly. Frequent adjustments to therapy may be required throughout the disease.

The treatment plan should clearly outline measurable goals like pain levels, morning stiffness duration, and physical abilities that indicate treatment efficacy. Patients should understand the plan's aims and share expectations with their healthcare team. Ongoing communication allows for adjusting therapy to meet evolving goals.

Optimal rheumatoid arthritis treatment improves daily well-being in both the short and long term by relieving symptoms, stemming joint damage, maximizing physical abilities, and striving for remission. No single goal takes primacy; combining approaches leads to the best outcomes.

Medications Used to Treat Rheumatoid Arthritis

Several medications help manage rheumatoid arthritis symptoms and progression. These include non-steroidal anti-inflammatory drugs (NSAIDs), disease-modifying anti-rheumatic drugs (DMARDs), biologic agents, corticosteroids, and analgesic pain relievers.

NSAIDs like ibuprofen, naproxen, and celecoxib provide analgesic and anti-inflammatory effects to ease joint pain and stiffness. They can help relieve symptoms but do not alter the progression of the disease. NSAIDs may be used alone for very mild cases or combined with other medications.

Disease-modifying anti-rheumatic drugs (DMARDs) such as methotrexate, hydroxychloroquine, and sulfasalazine can slow or stop the progression of rheumatoid arthritis and prevent joint damage. DMARDs suppress immune system activity, driving inflammation. Early DMARD treatment is key.

Biologic agents like adalimumab, etanercept, and infliximab are a newer class of DMARDs. They target specific inflammatory molecules or immune cells involved in rheumatoid arthritis. Biologics are used for moderate-to-severe rheumatoid arthritis that is unresponsive to conventional DMARDs alone.

Corticosteroids like prednisone directly combat inflammation. They can provide rapid, short-term relief during severe flares when taken orally, intravenously, or injected into joints. Long-term oral steroids have significant side effects.

Analgesics relieve joint pain symptoms. Over-the-counter options like acetaminophen provide mild pain relief. Prescription opioids or tramadol may be warranted temporarily for severe pain during flares when other treatments are inadequate.

Medications are often combined for synergistic effects. For example, a DMARD to modify disease progression can be paired with an NSAID for immediate pain relief or a biologic combination with methotrexate. Medications are adjusted over time to achieve remission.

Rheumatoid arthritis medications can cause side effects like nausea, increased infection risk, and liver toxicity that must be carefully managed through monitoring. Benefits and risks are weighed when selecting medications and combinations for each patient.

Treatment typically starts with one conventional DMARD, progressing to combinations or biologics depending on the initial response. Rapidly progressing, high-risk cases may begin with biologics and methotrexate. The goal is to induce remission and taper medications when possible.

In addition to medications, non-drug approaches like occupational therapy, splinting, and surgery provide multifaceted rheumatoid arthritis treatment. Complementary therapies further help manage symptoms and improve quality of life. There is no singular best protocol; rheumatologists personalize therapy based on each patient's unique disease course.

Lifestyle Approaches for Managing Rheumatoid Arthritis

Along with medications, certain lifestyle measures and therapies can help rheumatoid arthritis patients manage symptoms and preserve joint health. Recommended approaches include joint-friendly physical activity, joint protection techniques, eating an anti-inflammatory diet, occupational therapy, and surgery if needed.

Regular low-impact exercise provides numerous benefits for rheumatoid arthritis patients. Walking, swimming, cycling, and range-of-motion exercises improve joint mobility, strengthen supportive muscles, reduce pain, and improve mood. However, exercises should not further damage joints.

Joint protection techniques minimize the stress on damaged joints during daily tasks. Approaches include proper joint positioning, distributing weight evenly, avoiding staying in one position too long, using larger joints to perform movements when possible, and adaptive devices like jar openers.

An anti-inflammatory diet emphasizes fruits, vegetables, whole grains, and healthy fats like olive oil while limiting processed foods, sugar, excess salt, and saturated fats. This nutritional approach may help reduce joint inflammation. Omega-3 fatty acids also fight inflammation.

Occupational therapy helps patients adapt daily living activities like dressing, bathing, cooking, and driving to minimize joint stress and maximize function. Custom splints, mobility aids, and home modifications are often recommended.

Some patients undergo surgeries like synovectomy to remove inflamed joint linings, tendon reconstruction, or joint replacement if joint damage is severe. Surgery aims to repair deformities and restore maximal function, but it is inappropriate for all patients.

Quitting smoking is strongly advised, as it worsens rheumatoid inflammation and symptoms in multiple ways. Smoking cessation may slow disease progression. Stress management also helps control flares.

If warranted, a multidisciplinary approach combining medications, exercise, joint protection, nutrition, therapy, and surgery gives rheumatoid arthritis patients the best results. Lifestyle changes empower patients to self-manage their condition. Healthcare providers can recommend personalized programs.

While medications treat the disease, non-drug therapies and lifestyle approaches address the daily quality of life. Learning individual strategies to minimize joint strain and inflammation fosters independence and active participation in care. A holistic treatment plan improves well-being in both the short and long term.

Integrative Approaches Used for RA

In addition to standard medical therapies, some rheumatoid arthritis patients utilize integrative medicine to help manage symptoms and improve well-being. These complementary therapies include dietary supplements, mind-body practices, massage, and acupuncture.

Several nutritional supplements may provide anti-inflammatory effects and natural pain relief. These include omega-3 fish oils, turmeric/curcumin, ginger, *Gamma-Linoleic Acid* (GLA), pepperine, and marijuana-derived CBD oil. However, clinical evidence regarding efficacy and optimal dosing is still limited.

Mind-body therapies like meditation, yoga, tai chi, deep breathing, and guided imagery help counteract the stress of living with chronic illness. Relaxation techniques reduce muscle tension, anxiety, and depression while also lowering inflammatory responses that can worsen symptoms.

Massage therapy enhances relaxation, eases muscle tightness and joint stiffness, and improves mobility. Various massage methods can increase circulation, reduce swelling, and relieve natural pain by releasing endorphins.

Acupuncture involves inserting thin needles into specific body points to rebalance energy flow. Some patients report that acupuncture lessens arthritis pain and stiffness. It may work by tamping down inflammation and neural pain signaling.

Low-level laser therapy directs light energy of certain wavelengths into joints to stimulate tissue repair and suppress inflammation. Some patients notice reduced pain and swelling, but controlled studies are lacking.

Hydrotherapy involves exercising in warm water for cardiovascular benefits and easier joint mobility than land-based activity. The water's buoyancy minimizes joint stress.

Creams containing capsaicin from chili peppers provide topical pain relief by desensitizing nerve endings. However, they can irritate sensitive skin.

Wearing copper bracelets is another popular home remedy but with limited evidence.

While integrative therapies generally have few risks when used carefully, patients should discuss them with doctors to evaluate their appropriateness. They should not replace standard rheumatoid arthritis treatment. Additionally, larger studies are needed to confirm their usefulness and efficacy.

Some patients report that complementary approaches like yoga, massage, and acupuncture help enhance conventional treatment. However, individual responses vary. Rheumatologists can safely integrate approaches that improve patients' well-being into comprehensive care.

Chapter 5

Living with Rheumatoid Arthritis

Tips for Managing Common Rheumatoid Arthritis Symptoms

In addition to medical treatment, certain lifestyle measures and therapies can help rheumatoid arthritis patients better cope with troublesome symptoms like chronic pain, fatigue, and mobility impairment that affect daily life.

For pain management, over-the-counter analgesics, hot and cold therapy, distraction techniques, pacing activities, and mind-body practices such as meditation or yoga provide relief without the risks of long-term narcotic use. Setting a realistic pain control goal with your doctor is key.

Fatigue can be combated by getting adequate sleep, moderate exercise to boost energy, taking scheduled rests, eliminating unnecessary tasks, planning proper nutrition, and treating anemia or depression if present. Communicate with your employer about potential workplace accommodations.

Mobility challenges can be addressed through range-of-motion exercises, physical or occupational therapy, orthotics, and assistive devices, home modifications like grab bars, and learning proper joint protection techniques. Start slow and gradually increase activity.

Work with your healthcare team to find the right balance of medication, physical measures like splinting, complementary therapies like massage, and lifestyle adjustments tailored to manage your symptoms. Keep symptom journals to identify triggers and note what provides relief.

Pace yourself between activities by scheduling recuperation periods to avoid overexertion. Break up tasks into smaller, manageable steps. Listen to your body's signals and rest when needed. Let others know when you need assistance.

To reduce pain and stiffness:

- Apply heat before activities and ice packs after.
- Take warm baths and stretch gently.
- Use relaxation techniques, like deep breathing.
- Avoid staying in one position too long.
- Maintain good posture.

Minimize the load on joints during everyday tasks by using larger joints, keeping items within easy reach, and using assistive devices for grip and mobility. Distribute weight evenly and maintain muscle strength.

Nurture your emotional health through counseling, support groups, stress management, expressive arts, and spiritual practices. Stay engaged in fulfilling relationships and activities at your own pace. A positive outlook helps.

Explore supplementary therapies like massage, acupuncture, and dietary supplements. However, always discuss them with your rheumatologist first for safety. Do not disregard prescribed treatment.

With rheumatoid arthritis, flares and worsening of symptoms over time are expected. Tracking and managing symptoms is crucial in maximizing comfort and function. There are many tools to help you live well.

The Role of Physical and Occupational Therapy in Managing Rheumatoid Arthritis

Physical and occupational therapy provides invaluable tools for those with rheumatoid arthritis to help maintain strength, mobility, and independence in daily functioning.

Physical therapists design tailored exercise programs to improve muscle strength, joint flexibility, range of motion, balance, and aerobic fitness. They instruct patients on proper techniques for safe exercise without worsening joint damage. Aquatic therapy in warm pools is often utilized.

Stretching tight muscles around affected joints is a key focus of physical therapy. Gentle range-of-motion exercises reduce stiffness and prevent frozen joints. Light resistance training maintains supportive muscles while avoiding heavy joint loading.

Aerobic activity improves cardiovascular health, combats fatigue, and helps control weight. Exercises are selected based on disease activity and joint vulnerability. Walking, cycling, and swimming are frequent choices.

Physical therapists continuously monitor and adjust activity levels and exercises based on individuals' responses. They provide assistive devices like canes or splints as needed. Therapy goals center on sustained functionality.

Occupational therapists help patients devise ways to perform daily activities in joint-sparing ways. They instruct on the effective use of orthoses and mobility aids for specific challenges.

Strategies like distributing the load across multiple joints, using stronger joints to complete motions, and modifying tasks are taught. Seated positions for activities like bathing, dressing, and cooking are demonstrated to reduce strain.

Occupational therapists conduct home safety assessments to identify adaptations such as grab bars, raised toilets, and chair lifts that promote independent function. Recommendations help maximize independence.

Occupational therapy also improves joint protection during work. Workstation evaluations ensure proper positioning and ergonomics. Recommendations for assistive devices, schedule modifications, task swaps, or accommodations are given.

Both physical and occupational therapy empower patients with knowledge and skills for self-management. Patients take an active role in their care by learning techniques to safely preserve mobility and perform necessary daily tasks.

Assistive Devices That Can Help Patients with Rheumatoid Arthritis

Various assistive devices are available to aid rheumatoid arthritis patients in protecting vulnerable joints and maintaining independence in daily activities. Commonly used devices include splints, braces, canes, reaching aids, and adaptive equipment.

Splints are rigid supports worn on wrists, hands, fingers, elbows, ankles, or feet to immobilize and rest inflamed joints. They stabilize loose or damaged joints and prevent painful motion. Splints can be custom-fitted by occupational therapists.

Braces also provide joint support but allow some motion. Knee, wrist, ankle, and finger braces offer compression and stabilize alignment. Shoulder braces can assist movement in weakened shoulder joints. Neck braces support and restrict the motion of the cervical spine.

Canes transfer weight from lower extremity joints to the arms when walking, reducing pain and instability in knees, hips, ankles, and feet affected by arthritis. A physical therapist helps determine the proper cane size, shape, and walking technique.

Reaching aids like grab sticks enable picking up objects without excessive bending and strain on the back, shoulders, or fingers. Sock aids help avoid difficult hip and knee flexion when dressing. Long-handled sponges make bathing less taxing.

Jar openers, extended zipper pulls, large-handled utensils, wheeled carts, and other specialized tools take pressure off-hand joints when cooking, cleaning, and performing daily tasks. Built-up or extended handles decrease grip strain.

Adaptive equipment like raised toilet seats, shower chairs, mobility scooters, and bed rails help protect joints when transferring, bathing, and resting. Handles and banisters provide support on stairs. Sit-to-stand lifts aid standing.

Assistive technology offers computer options like speech recognition software and alternative mice or keyboards to accommodate limited hand functions.

Switches and environmental controls enable independent access.

Occupational therapists recommend devices tailored to each patient's capabilities and limitations. Proper use should be demonstrated to avoid other joint strains. Regular evaluation ensures aids continue meeting needs as arthritis progresses. Assistive devices promote self-sufficiency.

Though not appropriate for all patients, devices play important supportive roles in management. Braces, splints, or canes should complement, not replace, medical treatment and joint protection education. With guidance, aids provide functional assistance without fostering dependence.

The Psychological Impacts of Rheumatoid Arthritis and Healthy Coping Methods

Living with a chronic condition like rheumatoid arthritis frequently takes a psychological toll. Coping with pain, disability, medication side effects, and lifestyle limitations often leads to increased stress, depression, and anxiety in patients. Maintaining mental health is key.

It is very common to experience periods of frustration, sadness, fear, or hopelessness after an RA diagnosis or during disease flares. Restrictions in activity, independence, and career may necessitate difficult adjustments. Grief over these losses is normal.

In addition to emotional reactions, rheumatoid arthritis increases the risk of clinical depression and anxiety disorders. Chronic inflammation and immune activity in the brain, chronic pain, and drug therapies like steroids contribute to mood disorders.

Seeking professional counseling or peer support can help patients process difficult feelings and develop healthy coping mechanisms. Support groups connect individuals facing similar challenges. Stress management is important.

Prioritizing self-care through nourishment, restorative activities, relaxation techniques, and social connection counter the stresses of RA. Regular, moderate exercise boosts mental health. Adequate pain management aids in coping.

Mindfulness practices help regulate negative thoughts and emotions. Meditation, deep breathing exercises, yoga, and guided visualization calm the mind and body. Listening to music, reading, or the creative arts also provides outlets.

Redefining self-worth beyond disability or dependency is essential. Focus on remaining capable and valuable to loved ones. Be open about your needs so others can provide appropriate support. Save energy for meaningful activity.

While difficult, avoiding negative self-talk, catastrophizing, and rumination over unchangeable circumstances helps maintain positivity and purpose. Reframing setbacks as temporary and focusing on what you can control shifts perspective.

Professional or peer counseling aids in adjusting expectations, establishing new fulfilling routines and finding purpose in the face of physical limitations. Support builds resilience.

A proactive approach combining medication, healthy outlets for stress, strong social support, and cognitive-behavioral techniques fosters emotional well-being. With time and tools, people with RA can thrive despite physical challenges.

Pregnancy and Family Planning for Patients with Rheumatoid Arthritis

Rheumatoid arthritis poses some special considerations for pregnancy and family planning. With proper management, most women with RA can have healthy pregnancies and children.

Ideally, rheumatoid arthritis should be well-controlled for at least 3–6 months before attempting to conceive. Active disease raises the risk of complications and medication effects on the fetus. Achieving remission optimizes outcomes.

Most rheumatoid arthritis medications, like DMARDs, biologics, and NSAIDs, need to be stopped before conception due to potential fetal harm. Exceptions include the safe drugs hydroxychloroquine, sulfasalazine, low-dose prednisone, and some NSAIDs after the first trimester.

Before pregnancy, patients should discuss medication adjustments, nutrition, safe exercise, and monitoring with their rheumatologist. More frequent appointments monitor disease activity. Medications may be restarted after delivery.

Pregnancy hormone shifts often induce rheumatoid arthritis remission, especially in the second trimester. However, the first trimester and post-partum period tend to see flares as hormones fluctuate. Pain management without putting the baby at risk is important.

Women whose rheumatoid arthritis is active during pregnancy have a higher risk of complications, like premature birth. Babies may have mild, temporary symptoms after in-utero exposure to some medications. Breastfeeding is typically not recommended.

Partners should understand the risks of medications to sperm and the prospects of passing rheumatoid arthritis genes to children. Family planning should be thoughtfully discussed with the rheumatology team. Genetic counseling provides guidance.

During pregnancy, checkups monitor for preeclampsia, infection, osteoporosis, and other RA-related risks requiring intervention. Extended rest periods and modified activity are often advised.

Childbirth choices balance reduced strain on affected joints with delivery safety. Vaginal birth with epidural anesthesia avoids the risks of cesarean sections. Extended recovery times are expected.

Arthritis flares and fatigue make parenting young infants challenging. Having support from family, friends, and partners can be extremely beneficial during the post-partum period. It may be helpful to have assistance at home to provide some relief.

With prudent planning, advice from specialists, and adequate support, the majority of women with managed rheumatoid arthritis can safely navigate pregnancy and parenting challenges. A collaborative team effort optimizes outcomes.

Chapter 6

Associated Health Risks

Health Risks Associated with RA

In addition to joint symptoms and complications, rheumatoid arthritis increases the risk of several other significant health conditions, including cardiovascular disease, osteoporosis, infections, and certain cancers. Managing these associated health threats is an important aspect of comprehensive rheumatoid arthritis care.

1. **Cardiovascular Disease:** The chronic systemic inflammation of rheumatoid arthritis promotes atherosclerosis, the plaque buildup that narrows arteries and leads to heart attacks

and strokes. Patients have a nearly 50% higher risk of cardiovascular events compared to the general population. Regular screenings for cardiovascular risk factors are essential.

2. **Osteoporosis:** Bone loss is accelerated in rheumatoid arthritis, particularly around inflamed joints. The osteoporosis and bone density loss rate is two to four times higher among RA patients compared to healthy adults. Corticosteroid medications used to treat RA also contribute to this increased risk. Fractures often result, especially in the hip and spine.

3. **Infections:** The immunosuppressive medications used to treat rheumatoid arthritis raise patients' susceptibility to bacterial, viral, and fungal infections. Respiratory infections like pneumonia and influenza are common and serious. Septic arthritis stemming from joint injections is another potential concern requiring caution.

4. **Cancer:** Though uncommon, people with rheumatoid arthritis have a slightly elevated risk of developing certain cancers like

lymphoma and lung cancer over their lifetime. The increased cancer risk may be tied to immune system dysfunction and chronic inflammation. Some rheumatoid arthritis medications also potentially increase cancer vulnerability.

Screening and Preventive Care

In light of these associated health risks, close monitoring and preventive care are essential for rheumatoid arthritis patients. Recommended screenings include regular cardiovascular assessments, bone density scans, age-appropriate cancer screenings, and vaccination against preventable infections like pneumonia and influenza.

Prompt antibiotic treatment of infections is also key. Reducing other controllable risk factors, like smoking, is crucial as well. Rheumatologists and primary care physicians work together to provide comprehensive, multi-disciplinary care addressing the complex needs of rheumatoid arthritis patients. With proper management, the heightened risks can be minimized.

Cancer Screening Recommendations for Patients with Rheumatoid Arthritis

Due to immune dysfunction and chronic inflammation, people with rheumatoid arthritis have a moderately increased lifetime risk for certain cancers, especially lymphoma and lung cancer. Appropriate cancer screening allows for early detection and treatment in this higher-risk group.

General population screening guidelines apply to most rheumatoid arthritis patients, with a few additional considerations due to their elevated risk. Recommendations include:

1. **Breast Cancer:** Annual mammograms start at age 40 for average-risk women, with possible earlier screening for high-risk women. Inform radiology staff about rheumatoid arthritis and take precautions during positioning.

2. **Cervical Cancer:** Pap smears every 3–5 years for women aged 21–65. Some organizations prefer HPV testing with Pap smears.

Immunosuppression may increase HPV infection risk.

3. **Colorectal Cancer:** Colonoscopies every 10 years begin at age 45 for average-risk adults or earlier if high-risk factors exist. Some guidelines recommend starting regular screening at age 40 in rheumatoid arthritis patients due to higher risks.

4. **Skin Cancer:** Annual full-body skin exams by a dermatologist, with regular self-exams. A higher melanoma risk is linked to immunosuppressive medications in rheumatoid arthritis.

5. **Lymphoma:** No standard screening is available, but rheumatoid arthritis patients should report persistent fevers, night sweats, lumps, or swelling lasting over 2 weeks to their providers, as these may indicate lymphoma.

6. **Lung Cancer:** The USPSTF recommends annual lung cancer screening with low-dose CT scans for high-risk current and former heavy smokers ages 50–80. Rheumatoid arthritis

patients who smoke may start screening at age 50.

7. **Prostate Cancer:** Discuss prostate cancer screening with male healthcare providers. The decision to pursue PSA testing should be individualized based on risk factors and life expectancy.

In addition to screenings, reducing risk factors like smoking and alcohol use is imperative for rheumatoid arthritis patients. Those on biologics or high-dose steroids need extra vigilance for symptoms, as these medications raise infection and cancer risks. Report any persistent, suspicious symptoms promptly to providers.

While enhanced cancer screening does increase early detection, it also risks over-testing and over-diagnosis of non-harmful conditions. Patients should discuss the benefits and downsides of more intensive screening with their providers to make informed decisions aligned with their priorities and values.

Link Between RA, Periodontal Disease, and Potential Eye Problems in Patients

Periodontal Disease

There appears to be an association between rheumatoid arthritis and periodontal (gum) disease. People with rheumatoid arthritis have a higher gum disease prevalence than the general population. Severe gum disease is associated with more active rheumatoid arthritis.

The link may stem from shared risk factors between the two chronic inflammatory conditions, like smoking and diabetes. There are also some common susceptibility genes.

The bacteria involved in gum infections are suspected to trigger the abnormal autoimmune pathways that lead to rheumatoid arthritis in genetically susceptible individuals. This theory is being investigated.

Treating gum disease does not appear to improve rheumatoid arthritis symptoms. However, maintaining good oral hygiene and managing periodontal disease is still important to avoid potential impacts on RA disease activity.

Eye Problems

Up to 25% of rheumatoid arthritis patients develop some eye condition related to the disease. These include:

- **Dry eyes (Sjögren's)** - from inflammation damaging moisture-producing glands
- **Episcleritis** - inflammation of the outer eye tissue
- **Scleritis** - inflammation of the white part of the eye
- **Keratoconjunctivitis sicca** - dryness of the cornea and conjunctiva
- **Uveitis** - inflammation of the uvea, the middle eye layer

Eye inflammation is typically treated with steroid eye drops and needs prompt medical attention to avoid vision loss. Eye symptoms should be reported to a rheumatologist. Ophthalmologic exams are recommended periodically.

While not directly life-threatening, eye complications significantly impact the quality of life. Managing rheumatoid arthritis inflammation helps minimize eye disease risks. With regular eye care, vision can be preserved and discomfort prevented.

Important Vaccinations for RA Patients

Due to impaired immune function from the disease and immunosuppressive medications, people with rheumatoid arthritis are at increased risk of infection. Certain vaccinations are critical to help prevent potentially serious illnesses.

1. **Pneumococcal Vaccines:** Two vaccines protect against the bacteria that cause pneumonia and meningitis. Pneumovax 23 protects against 23 strains. It is given twice, 5 years apart, followed by a third dose at age 65. Prevnar 13 targets 13 strains and is given once.

2. **Influenza Vaccine:** The seasonal flu vaccine helps prevent influenza, a respiratory infection that can be particularly dangerous for rheumatoid arthritis patients. An annual flu

shot is recommended for all RA patients over 6 months old before peak flu season.

3. **Shingles Vaccine:** Shingles result from the reactivation of the chickenpox virus. Immunosuppressed rheumatoid arthritis patients are at higher risk for this painful rash and nerve infection. The recombinant shingles vaccine, Shingrix, is over 90% effective and given in two doses.

4. **Hepatitis Vaccines:** Hepatitis A and B vaccines protect against these viral liver infections. Some rheumatoid arthritis medications make hepatitis infections more likely or serious. Vaccination is recommended for those with risk factors.

5. **Tetanus Vaccine:** A tetanus booster shot containing the diphtheria and pertussis vaccines (Tdap) should be received every 10 years. People with rheumatoid arthritis are more susceptible to tetanus infection as they are prone to skin breaks, which is the primary entry point for the bacteria that causes tetanus.

6. **Travel Vaccines:** Patients traveling to certain destinations may need typhoid, cholera, yellow fever, rabies, or meningitis vaccines. Additional vaccines may be recommended based on the areas visited.

Vaccines like *Measles-Mumps-Rubella* (MMR), varicella, and the live shingles vaccine Zostavax should generally be avoided. However, killed or inactive vaccines are safe for rheumatoid arthritis patients when given under medical supervision.

Conclusion

Rheumatoid arthritis is a complex autoimmune condition requiring comprehensive management. However, with knowledge, proper treatment, and lifestyle adaptations, most patients can find ways to manage symptoms and live full, rewarding lives effectively.

This guide provides an in-depth overview of rheumatoid arthritis to empower patients and caregivers to take an active role in care. Key points to remember include:

- Seeking early diagnosis and treatment to limit joint damage. Monitoring symptoms and regular doctor follow-ups are crucial.

- Work closely with your rheumatologist to find the optimal medication regimen with minimal side effects for disease control.

- In addition to medications, lifestyle approaches like joint protection, exercise, diet, and stress reduction complement care. Explore options like occupational therapy.

- Listen to your body and be attuned to flare-ups or new symptoms requiring attention. Keep track of symptoms and communicate promptly with your healthcare team.

- Protect joints from further strain by learning proper movement mechanics, assistive devices, weight management, and ergonomic modifications.

- Develop a personalized program of activity pacing, rest, and stress relief to combat fatigue and pain. Seek support if emotional struggles arise.

- Take precautions to reduce the risks of infections, falls, osteoporosis, and cardiovascular disease associated with rheumatoid arthritis. Get recommended health screenings.

- Though rheumatoid arthritis cannot be cured, remission should be the goal. Patients can manage symptoms successfully with an individualized treatment plan and lifestyle adjustments while enjoying fulfilling lives.

- Remember, knowledge is power. The more you understand your condition, the better equipped you are to make informed care decisions and live well.

Rheumatoid arthritis requires patience and perseverance, but it does not have to define you. With the proper education, tools, and support, you can take charge of your health and maintain an active, positive outlook. This guide provides you with the information you need to do so.

Ongoing Rheumatoid Arthritis Research for Improved Treatments and Potential Cures

There is currently no cure for rheumatoid arthritis; ongoing research brings hope for better treatments and potential strategies to induce lasting remission or even permanently stop the abnormal autoimmune response that drives this condition.

Scientists continue investigating the complex interplay between genetic and environmental factors that mistakenly trigger the immune system to attack the joints in rheumatoid arthritis. Identifying these keys could unlock preventive strategies. Gene therapies may be able to correct genetic defects connected to RA.

Researchers also study biomarkers and diagnostic techniques for earlier and more accurate rheumatoid arthritis detection before joints become irreversibly damaged. Experimental blood tests and imaging methods may someday replace delayed diagnosis based on clinical presentation alone. Early, precise diagnosis enables early treatment.

Exciting progress is being made in novel medication therapies for rheumatoid arthritis as scientists better understand the underlying immune pathways. New classes of biological DMARDs target specific molecules that perpetuate inflammation and joint destruction with precision. Early studies suggest that combining complementary biologics may enhance RA remission.

Novel small-molecule DMARDs that can be taken orally or topically are also developing. These emerging immunomodulators may provide similar benefits as biologics with easier administration, fewer infections, and lower costs.

Gene therapies that allow the silencing of pro-inflammatory genes or enhance natural immune regulation are also on the horizon. Scientists are investigating techniques to repair, regenerate, or replace damaged joint tissues using stem cells, tissue engineering, and 3D printing. Such biological approaches may someday restore joint function.

While a definitive cure is likely still far off, the incredible pace of modern medical discovery gives hope. Each breakthrough takes us one step closer to unlocking the mysteries of rheumatoid arthritis and developing curative options. With time and continued research, the prospects for living well with rheumatoid arthritis will only improve.

Resources for Rheumatoid Arthritis Patients and Caregivers Seeking More Information

Rheumatoid arthritis is a complex condition that requires comprehensive self-education to manage effectively. Many excellent resources exist to help patients and caregivers learn more.

Patient Advocacy Organizations

The Arthritis Foundation (www.arthritis.org) provides extensive educational resources on rheumatoid arthritis and support programs. Their website offers information on disease basics, treatment options, lifestyle tips, stories from real patients, and local resources.

The American College of Rheumatology (www.rheumatology.org) has videos, treatment guidelines, clinical trial resources, and a finds-a-rheumatologist tool. They publish free patient education pamphlets.

Nonprofits like CreakyJoints, Arthritis Introspective, and CureArthritis provide online education, social networks, and other resources specifically for arthritis patients. These organizations combine medical expertise with patient perspectives.

Books/Publications

Johns Hopkins Arthritis Center publishes an excellent patient guide titled Living Well With Rheumatoid Arthritis. Several other patient-focused books offer knowledge on managing medications, pain, emotions, exercise, intimacy, nutrition, and work.

Patient websites, blogs, magazines like Arthritis Today, and even apps are other handy resources. However, ensure the sources are reputable. Stick to those endorsed by arthritis foundations and universities.

Healthcare Team

Your rheumatologist, primary care physician, nurses, and specialty therapists are invaluable resources. Come prepared with questions, and communicate openly about your challenges and treatment goals.

Consider having family and friends accompany you to appointments to absorb and recall information. Get copies of lab results, imaging reports, and clinical notes.

Support Networks

Online groups connect rheumatoid arthritis patients across geographical distances. Local, in-person support groups foster connections within communities. Arthritis foundations offer mentoring programs that pair patients with experienced volunteers. Connecting with others facing similar challenges provides support and ideas.

Rheumatoid arthritis education never stops. Continue learning and growing your understanding. Shared knowledge empowers patients to live full, active lives.

The Importance of an Early Diagnosis and Proactive Treatment

Early diagnosis and proactive treatment are crucial in managing rheumatoid arthritis (RA) effectively and preventing long-term joint damage and deformities.

Here are some reasons why early diagnosis and treatment are essential:

1. **Slowing Disease Progression:** Early treatment can help slow the progression of RA, preventing or minimizing joint damage and deformities. Studies have shown that early and aggressive treatment can lead to better outcomes, including improved joint function and quality of life.

2. **Managing Symptoms:** Early treatment can help manage the symptoms of RA, such as joint pain, stiffness, and fatigue, allowing individuals to maintain their daily activities and quality of life.

3. **Preventing Systemic Complications:** Early treatment can help prevent or manage the systemic complications of RA, such as cardiovascular disease, lung involvement, and osteoporosis, reducing the risk of long-term complications.

4. **Improving Treatment Response:** Early diagnosis and treatment can improve the

response to treatment, allowing for better disease control and reducing the need for more aggressive therapies later on.

5. **Reducing Healthcare Costs:** Early diagnosis and treatment can reduce healthcare costs associated with RA, including hospitalizations, surgeries, and long-term disability.

It is essential for individuals experiencing symptoms of RA to seek medical attention promptly and work closely with their healthcare providers to develop a comprehensive treatment plan. By taking a proactive approach to managing RA, individuals can improve their outcomes, reduce the risk of long-term complications, and ultimately improve their quality of life.

Appendices

Glossary of Key Terms

Here is a glossary of key terms related to rheumatoid arthritis (RA):

Autoimmune disease: A condition in which the body's immune system mistakenly attacks its tissues, leading to inflammation and potential damage to organs and tissues.

Cartilage: A tough, flexible tissue covering the ends of bones in a joint, providing cushioning and smooth movement.

Chronic inflammation: A persistent inflammatory response that can damage tissue and contribute to the development and progress of various diseases, including RA.

Deformity: A structural abnormality or distortion of a joint or body part, often resulting from chronic inflammation and joint damage in RA.

Joint: The point where two or more bones meet, allowing for movement and flexibility.

Pannus: An abnormal tissue in the synovium of joints affected by RA, contributing to joint damage and deformity.

Remission: A period during which the symptoms of RA are minimal or absent, often achieved through effective treatment.

Rheumatoid factor: An antibody often present in the blood of individuals with RA, indicating an autoimmune response.

Synovium: The lining of the joint that produces synovial fluid, which lubricates and nourishes the joint.

T-cells: A type of white blood cell that plays a key role in the immune response, including the response in RA.

Directory of Patient Support Organizations and Resources

Here is a directory of patient support organizations and resources for individuals living with rheumatoid arthritis (RA):

1. **Arthritis Foundation:** A national organization that provides resources, education, and support for individuals with arthritis, including RA. The Arthritis Foundation offers a range of programs and services, including support groups, educational materials, and advocacy efforts.

2. **CreakyJoints:** A patient-centered organization that provides support and resources for individuals with arthritis, including RA. CreakyJoints offers online support groups, educational materials, and advocacy efforts.

3. **National Rheumatoid Arthritis Society (NRAS):** A UK-based organization that provides support and resources for individuals with RA. NRAS offers various services,

including a helpline, online forums, and educational materials.

4. **Rheumatoid Arthritis Support Network (RASN):** A patient-centered organization that provides support and resources for individuals with RA. RASN offers online support groups, educational materials, and advocacy efforts.

5. **American College of Rheumatology (ACR):** A professional organization that provides resources and education for healthcare providers and patients with rheumatic diseases, including RA. The ACR offers patient education materials, advocacy efforts, and a directory of rheumatologists.

6. **Healthline:** A website that provides information and resources on various health conditions, including RA. Healthline offers articles, videos, and tools to help individuals with RA manage their condition and improve their quality of life.

7. **Mayo Clinic:** A healthcare organization that provides information and resources on various health conditions, including RA. Mayo Clinic

offers articles, videos, and tools to help individuals with RA manage their condition and improve their quality of life.

By utilizing these patient support organizations and resources, individuals with RA and their caregivers can access valuable information, emotional support, and practical advice for managing RA and its impact on daily life.

www.ingramcontent.com/pod-product-compliance
Lightning Source LLC
Chambersburg PA
CBHW060944260726
48661CB00005B/1751